The Ultimate Guide to Dash Diet Meals for Everyone

Mesmerizing Healthy Snacks and Desserts for Busy People on Diet

I0135220

Naomi Hudson

Table of contents

Peanut Butter Sandwich Snacks

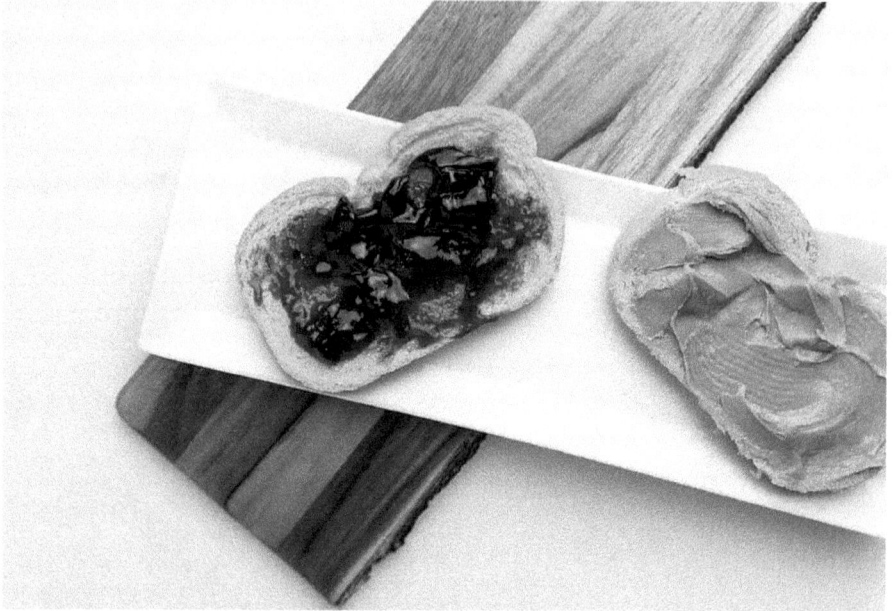

SmartPoints value: Green plan - 3SP, Blue plan - 3SP, Purple plan - 3SP

Total Time: 5 min, Prep time: 5 min, Serves: 1

Nutritional value: Calories - 327, Carbs - 30g, Fat - 17.9g, Protein - 15.0g

When you're looking for something sweet, chocolaty, and rich in nutrients, this easy-to-make snack will do the job. I make use of chocolate syrup as an alternative to melted chocolate. I observed that chocolate syrup has fewer Smart Points, and the small amount spreads farther. I should let you know that the chocolate syrup will not get hard, even when you refrigerate.

Ingredients

- Peanut butter (powdered) - 1 Tbsp

- Water - 2¼ tsp

- Crispbread, Whole Grain (34 degrees) - 6 crackers, or similar product

- Chocolate syrup - 1½ tsp

- Sprinkles - ¼ tsp, nonpareil

Instructions

1.   Mix the powdered peanut butter and water in a clean small bowl and stir until it becomes smooth.

2.   Spread the peanut butter evenly over three crackers and top it with the remaining three crackers biscuit or bread.

3.   Take half a teaspoon of chocolate syrup and spread it over half the top of each cracker sandwich — top chocolate syrup with sprinkles.

Peanut Butter Apple Slices

SmartPoints value: Green plan - 4SP, Blue plan - 4SP, Purple plan - 4SP

Total time: 10 min, Prep time: 10 min, Serves: 4

Nutritional value: Calories - 218, Carbs – 31.3g, Fat – 8.1g, Protein – 11.6g

Having a healthy snack ready in about 10 minutes is a thing of joy for me. Peanut butter apple slices are just what fits into the picture of a healthy quick, nutritious snack. This apple slice is a simple and easy meal rich in protein and fiber. It is topped with peanut butter and decorated with chocolate chips and slivered almonds.

Ingredients

- Large apples - 2 pieces

- Powdered peanut butter (reconstituted) - 1/2 cup

- Semi-sweet chocolate chips - 2 tbsp

- Slivered almonds - 2 tbsp

- Pecans (chopped) - 2 tbsp

Instructions

1.   Remove the core of the apple using a small paring knife or an apple corer

2.   Slice the apples into thick rings.

3.   Add the peanut butter on the apple slices.

4.   Use chips and nuts for top-up

Baked Plantains

SmartPoints value: Green plan - 5SP, Blue plan - 5SP, Purple plan - 5SP

Total time: 40 min, Prep time: 5 min, Cooking time: 35min, Serves: 2

Nutritional value: Calories - 184, Carbs - 47g, Fat – 0.5g, Protein - 2g

Baked plantain is just as healthy as it is tasty. The plantain is full of good for your ingredients.

Ingredients

- Very overripe plantains (2 medium-sized)

- Misting spray (Olive oil)

- Salt to taste

Instructions

1.   On a preheated oven of 350 degrees, line a baking sheet with a silicone mat or parchment paper and spray with olive oil or non-fat cooking spray.
2.   Thinly slice plantains and place them on the baking sheet evenly, then lightly mist with olive oil or the non-fat cooking spray and sprinkle with a bit of salt.

3.　　For about 30-35 minutes, cook in the oven flipping once about halfway through until they become golden and mostly crisp.

Baked plantains are easy to prepare and very firm. They taste sweeter when overly ripe, and firmer when they are not as ripe. Feel free to choose your style of plantain.

Strawberries & Cream Chocolate Cookie Sandwich

SmartPoints value: Green plan - 3SP, Blue plan - 3SP, Purple plan - 3SP

Total time: 5 min, Prep time: 5 min, Serves: 1

Nutritional value: Calories - 280, Carbs - 37g, Fat - 12g, Protein - 5g

I'm sure you will love this tasty summer treat. This chocolate cookie sandwich will remind you of your favorite childhood ice cream sandwich. This version is healthier, upgraded, and way easier to make in your kitchen! You can impress your loved ones with this delicious dessert/snack by making dozens of them for parties, barbecues, or special occasions with family and friends. If you don't have strawberries, you can substitute with any ripe fruit you have on hand like peaches, bananas, or raspberries.

Ingredients

- Topping (lite whipped) - 2 Tbsp Strawberries (hulled, sliced) - 1 medium

- Graham cracker(s) (chocolate variety) - 2 square(s)

Instructions

1.   Scoop whipped topping onto one square-shaped graham cracker.

2.   Top it with sliced strawberries and place another cracker on top of that.

Mini chocolate chip cookies

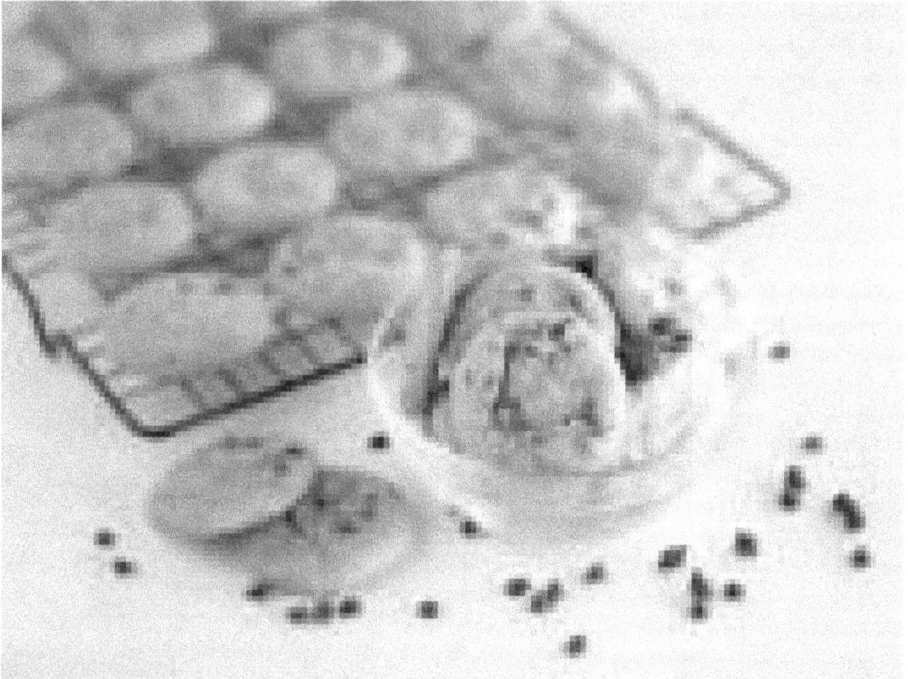

SmartPoints value: Green plan - 1SP, Blue plan - 1SP, Purple plan - 1SP

Total time: 26 min, Prep time: 10 min, Cooking time: 6 min, Serves: 48

Nutritional value: Calories - 113.7, Carbs - 16.4g, Fat - 5.9g, Protein - 0.6g

These bite-size cookies might be small, but they pack a chocolate punch. I often use dark brown sugar in making these cookies as it contains more molasses than the light brown variety. The dark brown sugar adds a rich, complex flavor to these cookies, making them moist and chewy. In case you have only light brown sugar available, you don't have to go out of your way to get the dark variety. That will work just fine. You can replace the chocolate chips with any other one you like, be it cinnamon chips, toffee, butterscotch, or white chocolate chips. You can even stir in some chopped nuts to make things a little cDashchy.

Ingredients

- Butter (salted, softened) - 2 Tbsp

- Canola oil - 2 tsp

- Brown sugar (packed, dark-variety) - ½ cup(s)

- Vanilla extract - 1 tsp

- Table salt - ⅛ tsp

- Egg white(s) - 1 large

- All-purpose flour - ¾ cup(s)

- Baking soda - ¼ tsp

- Chocolate chips (semi-sweet) - 3 oz, about 1/2 cup

Instructions

1.   Prepare the oven by preheating it to 375°F.

2.   Mix the butter, oil, and sugar in a medium bowl.
3.   Add vanilla and egg white, then mix thoroughly to combine. Toss in some salt to taste.
4.   Mix the flour and baking soda in a small bowl and stir them into the batter.
5.   Add the chocolate chips to the batter and stir to distribute evenly throughout.
6.   Put forty-eight half-teaspoons of dough onto two large nonstick baking sheets. Leave small spaces between the cookies.
7.   Bake the cookies until they become golden around the edges; about 4 to 6 minutes.
8.   Cool the baked cookies on a wire rack.

Chocolate-Peppermint Thins

SmartPoints value: Green plan - 3SP, Blue plan - 3SP, Purple plan - 3SP

Total Time: 1hr 16 min, Prep time: 15 min, Cooking time: 5 min, Serves: 16

Nutritional value: Calories - 175, Carbs – 21g, Fat – 5g, Protein – 7g

My homemade chocolate peppermint thin comes with a splash of peppermint extract, and divine copycat thin mint cookies to satisfy my cravings

Ingredients

- Chocolate chunk (coarsely chopped) - 3½ oz

- Chocolate wafer(s) (thin variety) - 16 item(s)

- Candy cane (finely crushed) - 1 oz

Instructions

1. Arrange a large baking sheet with parchment or paper wax and line cookies close together in a single layer.

2. At 5 seconds interval, melt chocolate in a microwavable bowl and stir between each interval until all but one or two pieces

melted, then remove from microwave and stir until fully dissolved.

3.	Put the melted chocolate in a plastic bag and cut off a corner; in a zig-zag pattern, pipe the chocolate over cookies and sprinkle with the crushed candy cane, keep it refrigerated until its set for at least

an hour or overnight. Serve as desired (1 cookie per serving)

Chocolate-Dipped Baby Bananas

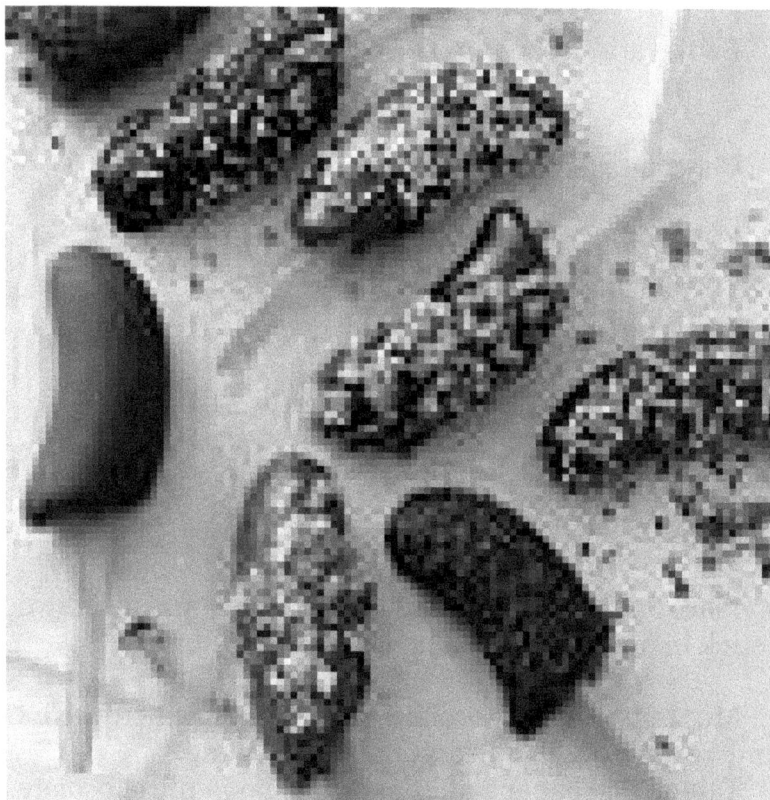

SmartPoints value: Green plan - 3SP, Blue plan - 3SP, Purple plan - 3SP

Total time: 20 min, Prep time: 5 min, Cooking time: --, Serves: 12

Nutritional value: Calories - 210, Carbs – 31.2g, Fat – 1g, Protein – 5.4g

Chocolate-dipped baby bananas are just perfect for casual parties for both kids and adults. With the banana and chocolate combination, it's so irresistible. Alternatively, you can replace baby bananas with four regular bananas cut crosswise into thirds.

Ingredients

- Baby-variety banana (peeled) - 12 small

- Chocolate (semisweet, chopped) - 3 oz

- Butter (unsalted) - ¾ tsp

- Coconut (shredded, unsweetened) - 2 tbsp

Instructions

1.   Place large baking sheet with wax paper and insert wooden craft stick in one end of each banana.

2.   Mix butter and chocolate in a medium microwave bowl, then microwave on high heat for about 1minute.
3.   Taking one banana after another spoon the chocolate over the bananas cover, and sprinkle it with coconut while it is on a baking sheet. Keep it refrigerated until the chocolate sets in about 15 minutes.
4.   Serve as desired (1 banana per serving)

Fall Harvest Salad

SmartPoints value: Green plan - 3SP, Blue plan - 1SP, Purple plan - 1SP

Total time: 15 min, Prep time: 15 min, Cooking time: 0 min, Serves: 4

Nutritional value: Calories - 175, Carbs – 25.7g, Fat – 7.6g, Protein – 4.8g

Whether or not you have planned for a holiday meal, this fall harvest salad

will fire up some inspiration, and get those juices flowing.

If this would be your first time giving this a try, I trust you'll be looking for excuses to make this salad over and over again.

There are two most seen together in desserts, that's the flavor combination of cinnamon and apples. They both make undeniable mouthwatering delicious flavors in this fall harvest salad.

I also love to add some Honey crisp apples (my favorite apple), or sometimes I use Fuji, a pink lady on this Harvest Salad. They all blend well.

To prevent my apples from getting brown after slicing, I avoid exposing it to air. When the apples turn brown, your salad would not be as pretty as you would love it. I will add a little, so that will help you avoid this problem and keep your apples beautiful

After slicing your apple, submerge the slices in a bowl of saltwater (I usually mix about 1 tbsp of salt with 1 ½ cups of water) then stir it until the salt dissolves then add in the apple slices. Let it sit for about 5 minutes and then rinse the slices with water and pat dry with a paper towel.

That's just it. So simple, yeah? This way of cutting apples has been working for me for ages, and I love it more because it's cheaper and cleaner than buying those bags of pre-cut apples.

Ingredients

- Kale greens (baby variety) - 4-5 cups

- Large apple (thinly sliced) - 1 piece

- Sweet pumpkin seeds (toasted) - 1/3 cup

For dressing

- Olive oil - 1 tbsp

- Maple Syrup - 1 tbsp

- Red wine vinegar - 2 tbsp

- Shallot (minced) - 1 piece

- Cinnamon - ¼ tsp

- Dijon mustard - 1 tsp

- Pepper and salt to taste

Instructions

1.   Beat all the ingredients for the dressing together in a small bowl

2.   Toss the ingredients for the salad in a large bowl
3.   Pour the processed dressing over the salad and toss to coat evenly

4.   This perfect dish is sure to impress your guests and compliment your holiday meal. Be careful not to lick the bowl.

Mediterranean Baked Tilapia

SmartPoints value: Green plan - 3SP, Blue plan - 1SP, Purple plan - 1SP

Total time: 25 min, Prep time: 10 min, Cooking time: 15 min, Serves: 4

Nutritional value: Calories - 129, Fat - 5g, Protein - 21g

During festive periods, it gets more tempting to eat just every meal that crosses by you. That's why I'm creating this recipe to help you maintain low SP meals during those periods. Let's take a look at the deliciously outlined recipe.

Ingredients

- Tilapia fillets - 1 lb (about eight fillets)

- Olive oil - 1 tsp

- Butter - 1 tbsp

- Shallots (finely chopped) - 2 pieces

- Garlic (minced) - 3 cloves

- Cumin (ground) - 1 1/2 tsp

- Paprika (1 1/2 tsp)

- Capers (1/4 cup)

- Dill (finely chopped, fresh) - 1/4 cup

- Lemon juice - from 1 lemon

- Pepper and salt to taste

Instructions

1.   Line a rimmed baking sheet with parchment paper or foil over a preheated oven of 375 degrees. Mist with cooking spray and spread fish fillets evenly on the baking sheet.
2.   Combine the paprika, pepper, and salt in a small bowl. Season the fish fillets with the spice mixture on both sides.
3.   Whisk together in a small bowl, the melted butter, olive oil, lemon juice, shallots, and garlic then brush evenly over the fish fillets.

Top with the capers.

4.   Making sure not to overcook, bake in the oven for about 10-15 minutes, then remove from oven and top with fresh dill.

Two-Ingredient Ice Cream Cupcake Bites

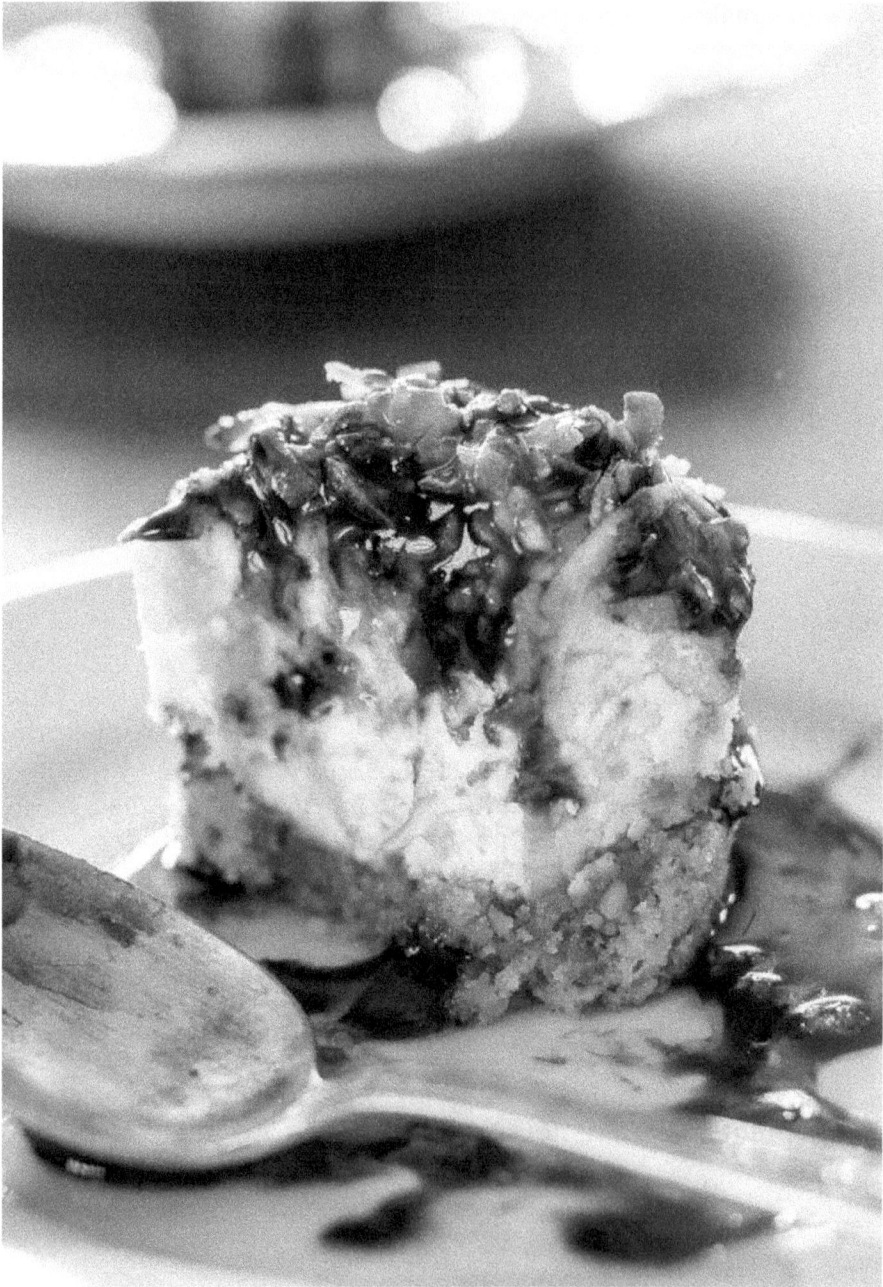

SmartPoints value: Green plan - 2SP, Blue plan - 2SP, Purple plan - 2SP

Total Time: 32 min, Prep time: 5 min, Cooking time: 12 min, Serves: 12

Nutritional value: Calories - 109, Carbs - 10g, Fat - 8g, Protein - 12g

You won't get any fresh-baked dessert or snack that is easier or more lovely than these two-ingredient mini cupcakes. All it takes is to mash your favorite

WW ice cream bars and combine with self-rising flour, then bake it. You can eat it as it is or finish it off with whipped topping and sprinkles. They are perfect for birthday parties, snacks, and more.

Ingredients

- Ice cream bars (WW Dark Chocolate-raspberry) - 6 bar(s) White flour (self-rising) - 10 Tbsp Whipped topping (light) - 4 Tbsp Sprinkles (rainbow) - ½ Tbsp

Instructions

1.   After preheating the oven to 350°F, coat twelve mini muffin holes with cooking spray

2.   Drop the ice cream from the sticks into a large bowl and allow it to melt slightly, then add some white flour and stir until it is well-mixed.

3.   Evenly fill prepared muffin holes with the mixture and bake until a tester inserted in the center of a cupcake comes out without anything sticking to it; about 10-12 minutes.

4. Allow the cupcakes to cool in the pan for a few minutes before taking them out. Collect the processed muffins from the pan and cool completely.

5. Put one teaspoon of whipped topping in each cooled cupcake and divide the sprinkles over the top.

Lemon Blueberry Cheesecake Yogurt Bark

SmartPoints value: 1SP

Total time: 1 hr 15 mins, Prep time: 15 mins, Chill time: 1 hr, Serves - 12

Nutritional value: Calories - 124, Carbs - 12.7g, Fat - 0.2g, Protein - 18.2g

Ingredients

- Greek yogurt (plain non-fat) - 1 cup

- Agave nectar - 1 tablespoon

- Lemon zest - 1/2 teaspoon

- Lemon juice (fresh-squeezed) - 1/2 teaspoon Blueberries (fresh) - 1 cup

- Graham crackers (crushed into crumbs) - 3 squares (gluten-free if you like)

Instructions

1.   Line a 9x5-inch loaf pan with aluminum foil so that the foil hangs over sides of the pan.

2.   Mix the yogurt, lemon zest, agave nectar, and lemon juice in a small mixing bowl, then stir.

3.   Turn in the blueberries gently with three tablespoons crushed graham cracker crumbs just until adequately mixed.

4.   Evenly spread the mixture into the loaf pan you earlier prepared. Get the remaining cracker crumbs and sprinkle over the top.

5.   Use aluminum foil to cover the loaf pan and refrigerate for at least 1 hour; until it is frozen.

6.   Once the mixture is frozen, remove the pan from the freezer and use overhanging foil as handles to lift the bark from the pan.

7.   Put the frozen mixture on a cutting board and slice it into eight squares.

8.   Cut each square diagonally, creating two triangles. (If the frozen dough is too difficult to cut, allow it to sit out at room temperature to soften. Alternatively, you can keep the knife inside hot water before cutting.)

9.   Keep the cut portions in an airtight container inside the freezer until you are ready to serve. Allow the cut triangles to sit on the table at room temperature to soften slightly before serving if it is too frozen

Dark Chocolate Avocado Mousse

This chocolate delicacy, loaded with healthy fats, fiber, and antioxidants, is a perfect dessert recipe.

SmartPoints value - 9SP

Total time: 1 hr 10 mins, Prep time: 10 mins, Chill time: 1 hr, Serves: 2

Nutritional value: Calories - 434, Carbs - 53g, Fat - 29g, Protein - 6g

Ingredients

- Avocado (very ripe, peeled and seeded) - 1 large

- Dark baking chocolate (70% cacao, melted) - 2 ounces

- Cocoa powder (unsweetened) - 2 Tbsp

- Almond milk (unsweetened) - 1/4 cup

- Maple syrup - 2 Tbsp

- Pure vanilla extract - 1/4 Tsp

- Cinnamon (ground) - A pinch

- Salt - A pinch

Instructions

1.   Get a blender and put in avocado, maple syrup, melted chocolate, milk, cocoa powder, vanilla, cinnamon, and salt.

2.   Process the content of the blender until you get a smooth and creamy mixture. To make the mousse thinner, add more milk or less milk for a thicker mousse.
3.   Pour the mixture evenly into two small dessert glasses.
4.   Chill it for at least 1 hour in the refrigerator before serving.

Hearty Chia and Blackberry Pudding

Serving: 2

Prep Time: 45 minutes

Cook Time: Nil

Ingredients:

- ¼ cup chia seeds

- ½ cup blackberries, fresh

- 1 teaspoon liquid sweetener

- 1 cup coconut almond milk, full fat and unsweetened

- 1 teaspoon vanilla extract

How To:

1.   Take the vanilla, liquid sweetener and coconut almond milk and add to blender.

2.   Process until thick.
3.   Add in blackberries and process until smooth.
4.   Divide the mixture between cups and chill for 30 minutes.
5.   Serve and enjoy!

Nutrition (Per Serving)

Calories: 437

Fat: 38g

Carbohydrates: 8g

Protein: 8g

Special Cocoa Brownie Bombs

Serving: 12

Prep Time: 15 minutes

Cooking Time: 25 minutes

Freeze Time: None

Ingredients:

- 2 tablespoons grass-fed almond butter

- 1 whole egg

- 2 teaspoons vanilla extract

- ¼ teaspoon baking powder

- 1/3 cup heavy cream

- 3/4 cup almond butter

- ¼ cocoa powder

- A pinch of sunflower seeds

How To:

1.   Break the eggs and whisk until smooth.

2.   Add in all the wet ingredients and mix well.
3.   Make the batter by mixing all the dry ingredients and sifting them into the wet ingredients.
4.   Pour into a greased baking pan.
5.   Bake for 25 minutes at 350 degrees F or until a toothpick inserted in the middle comes out clean.
6.   Let it cool, slice and serve.

Nutrition (Per Serving)

Total Carbs: 1g

Fiber: 0g

Protein: 1g

Fat: 20g

Gentle Blackberry Crumble

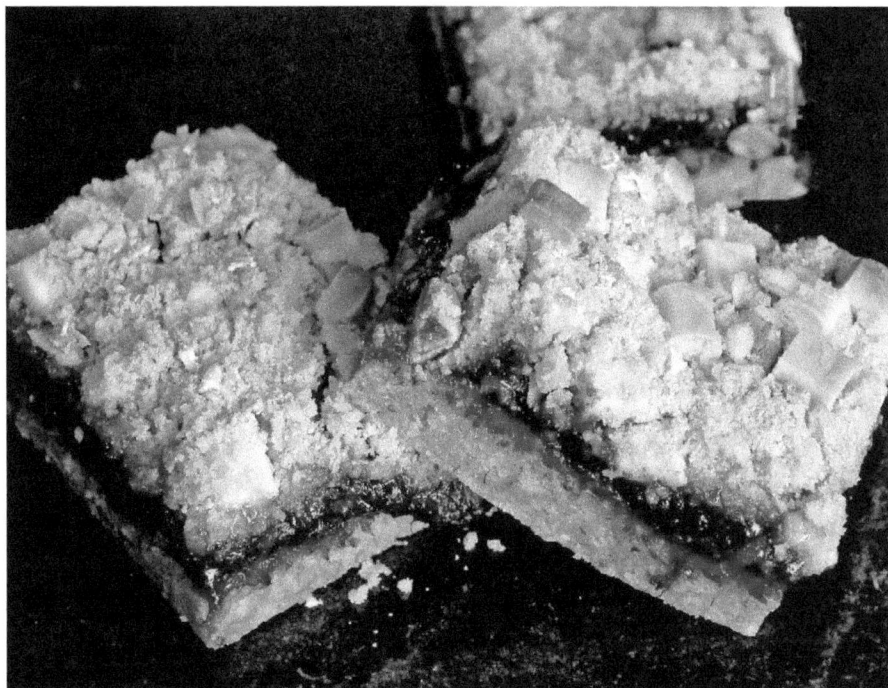

Serving: 4

Prep Time: 10 minutes

Cook Time: 45 minutes

Smart Points: 4

Ingredients:

- ½ cup coconut flour

- ½ cup banana, peeled and mashed

- 6 tablespoons water

- 3 cups fresh blackberries

- ½ cup arrowroot flour

- 1 ½ teaspoons baking soda

- 4 tablespoons almond butter, melted

- 1 tablespoon fresh lemon juice

How To:

1.   Pre-heat your oven to 300 degrees F.

2.   Take a baking dish and grease it lightly.
3.   Take a bowl and mix all of the ingredients except the blackberries, mix well.
4.   Place blackberries in the bottom of your baking dish and top with flour.
5.   Bake for 40 minutes.
6.   Serve and enjoy!

Nutrition (Per Serving)

Calories: 12

Fat: 7g

Carbohydrates: 10g

Protein: 4g

Mini Minty Happiness

Serving: 12

Prep Time: 45 minutes

Cooking Time: None Freeze Time: 2 hours

Ingredients:

- 2 teaspoons vanilla extract

- 1 ½ cups coconut oil

- 1 ¼ cups sunflower seed almond butter ½ cup dried parsley

- 1 teaspoon peppermint extract

- A pinch of sunflower seeds

- 1 cup dark chocolate chips Stevia to taste

How To:

1.   Melt together coconut oil and dark chocolate chips over a double boiler.

2.   Take a food processor, add all the ingredients into it and pulse until

smooth.

3.   Pour into round molds.

4.   Let it freeze.

Nutrition (Per Serving)

Total Carbs: 7g

Fiber: 1g

Protein: 3g

Fat: 25g

Astonishing Maple Pecan Bacon Slices

Serving: 12

Prep Time: 10 minutes

Cooking Time: 25 minutes

Freeze Time: None

Ingredients:

- tablespoon sugar-free maple syrup

- 12 bacon slices

- Granulated Stevia to taste

- 15-20 drops Stevia For the coating:

- 4 tablespoons dark cocoa powder

- ¼ cup pecans, chopped

- 15-20 drops Stevia

How To:

1.   Take a baking tray and lay the bacon slices on it.

2.   Rub with maple syrup and Stevia, flip the slices and do the same with the other side.
3.   Bake for 10-15 minutes at 227 degrees F.
4.   After they've baked, drain the bacon grease.
5.   To form a batter, mix the bacon grease, Stevia and cocoa powder.

6.   Dip the bacon slices into the batter and roll in the chopped pecans.

7.   Allow to air dry until the chocolate hardens.

Nutrition (Per Serving)

Total Carbs: 1g

Fiber: 0g

Protein: 10g

Fat: 11g

Generous Maple and Pecan Bites

Serving: 12

Prep Time: 10 minutes

Cooking Time: 25 minutes

Freeze Time: None

Ingredients:

- 1 cup almond meal

- ½ cup coconut oil

- ½ cup flaxseed meal

- ½ cup sugar-free chocolate chips

- 2 cups pecans, chopped

- ½ cup sugar-free maple syrup

- 20-25 drops Stevia

How To:

1.   Take a baking dish and spread the pecans.

2.   Bake at 350 degrees F until aromatic.
3.   This will usually take from 6 to 8 minutes.
4.   Meanwhile, sift together all the dry ingredients.
5.   Add the roasted pecans to the mix and mix them properly.
6.   Add the coconut oil and maple syrup.
7.   Stir to make a thick, sticky mixture.
8.   Take a bread pan lined with parchment paper, and pour the mixture into it.
9.   Bake for about 18 minutes.
10.   Slice and serve.

Nutrition (Per Serving)

Total Carbs: 6g

Fiber: 0g

Protein: 5g

Fat: 30g

Carrot Ball Delight

Serving: 4

Prep Time: 10 minutes

Cook Time: Nil

Ingredients:

- 6 Medjool dates pitted

- 1 carrot, finely grated

- ¼ cup raw walnuts

- ¼ cup unsweetened coconut, shredded

- 1 teaspoon nutmeg

- 1/8 teaspoon sunflower seeds

How To:

1.   Take a food processor and add dates, ¼ cup of grated carrots, sunflower seeds coconut, nutmeg.

2. Mix well and puree the mixture.
3. Add the walnuts and remaining ¼ cup of carrots.
4. Pulse the mixture until you have a chunky texture.
5. Form balls using your hand and roll them up in coconut.
6. Top with carrots and chill.
7. Enjoy!

Nutrition (Per Serving)

Calories: 326

Fat: 16g

Carbohydrates: 42g

Protein: 3g

Awesome Brownie Muffins

Serving: 5

Prep Time: 10 minutes

Cooking Time: 35 minutes

Ingredients:

1 cup golden flaxseed meal

- ¼ cup cocoa powder

- 1 tablespoon cinnamon

- ½ tablespoon baking powder

- ½ teaspoon sunflower seeds

- 1 whole large egg

- 2 tablespoons coconut oil

- ¼ cup sugar-free caramel syrup

- ½ cup pumpkin puree

- 1 teaspoon vanilla extract

- 1 teaspoon apple cider vinegar

- ¼ cup almonds, slivered

How To:

1.   Pre-heat your oven to 350 degrees F.

2.   Take a mixing bowl and add all of the listed ingredients and mix everything well.
3.   Take your desired number of muffin tins and line them with paper liners.
4.   Scoop the batter into the muffin tins, filling them to about 1/4 of the liner.
5.   Sprinkle a bit of almond on top.
6.   Place them in your oven and bake for 15 minutes.
7.   Serve warm.

Nutrition (Per Serving)

Total Carbs: 16

Fiber: 2g

Protein: 3g

Fat: 31g

Spice Friendly Muffins

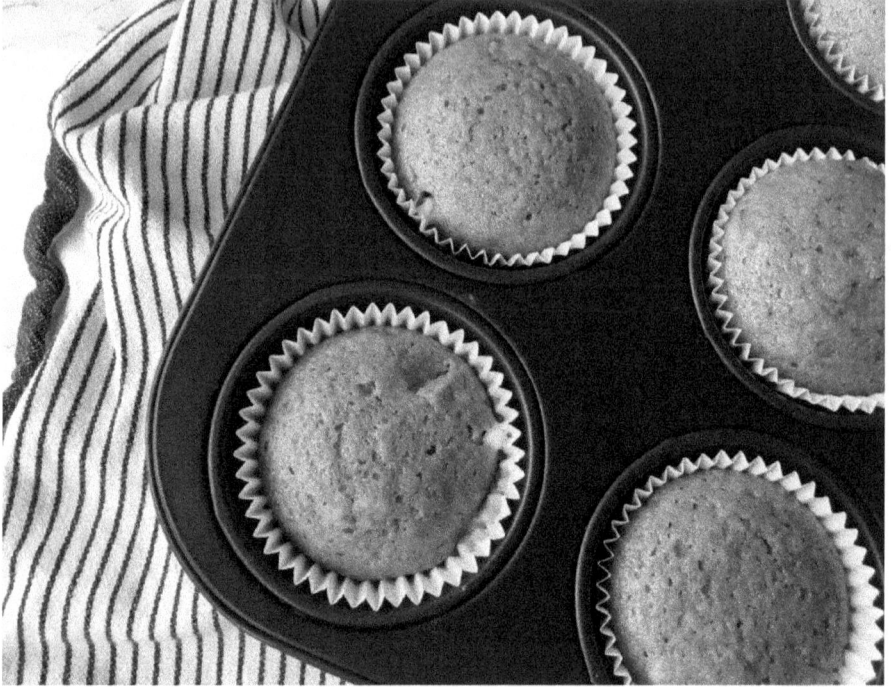

Serving: 12

Prep Time: 5 minutes

Cooking Time: 45minute

Ingredients:

- ½ cup raw hemp hearts

- ½ cup flaxseeds

- ¼ cup chia seeds

- 2 tablespoons Psyllium husk powder

- 1 tablespoon cinnamon

- Stevia taste

- ½ teaspoon baking powder

- ½ teaspoon sunflower seeds

- 1 cup of water

How To:

1. Pre-heat your oven to 350 degrees F.

2. Line muffin tray with liners.
3. Take a large sized mixing bowl and add peanut almond butter, pumpkin, sweetener, coconut almond milk, flaxseed and mix well.

4. Keep stirring until the mixture has been thoroughly combined.

5. Take another bowl and add baking powder, spices and coconut flour.
6. Mix well.

7.   Add the dry ingredients into the wet bowl and stir until the coconut flour has mixed well.

8.   Allow it to sit for a while until the coconut flour has absorbed all of the moisture.

9.   Divide the mixture amongst your muffin tins and bake for 45 minutes.

10.   Enjoy!

Nutrition (Per Serving)

Total Carbs: 7g

Fiber: 3g

Protein: 6g

Fat: 15g

Simple Gingerbread Muffins

Serving: 12

Prep Time: 5 minutes

Cooking Time: 30 minutes

Ingredients:

- 1 tablespoon ground flaxseed

- 6 tablespoons coconut almond milk

- 1 tablespoon apple cider vinegar

- ½ cup peanut almond butter

- 2 tablespoons gingerbread spice blend

- 1 teaspoon baking powder

- 1 teaspoon vanilla extract

- 2 tablespoons Swerve

How To:

1.   Pre-heat your oven to 350 degrees F.

2.   Take a bowl and add flaxseeds, sweetener, sunflower seeds, vanilla, spices and your non-dairy almond milk.
3.   Keep it on the side for a while.
4.   Add peanut almond butter, baking powder and keep mixing until combined well.
5.   Stir in peanut almond butter and baking powder.
6.   Mix well.
7.   Spoon the mixture into muffin liners.
8.   Bake for 30 minutes.
9.   Allow them to cool and enjoy!

Nutrition (Per Serving)

Total Carbs: 13g

Fiber: 4g

Protein: 11g

Fat: 23g

Fantastic Cauliflower Bagels

Serving: 12

Prep Time: 10 minutes

Cooking Time: 30 minutes

Ingredients:

- 1 large cauliflower, divided into florets and roughly chopped

- ¼ cup nutritional yeast

- ¼ cup almond flour

- ½ teaspoon garlic powder

- 1 ½ teaspoon fine sea sunflower seeds

- 1 whole egg

- 1 tablespoon sesame seeds

How To:

1. Pre-heat your oven to 400 degrees F.

2. Line a baking sheet with parchment paper, keep it on the side.

3. Blend cauliflower in the food processor and transfer to a bowl.

4. Add nutritional yeast, almond flour, garlic powder and sunflower seeds to a bowl, mix.
5. Take another bowl and whisk in eggs, add to cauliflower mix.
6. Give the dough a stir.
7. Incorporate the mix into the egg mix.
8. Make balls from dough, making a hole using your thumb into each ball.
9. Arrange them on your prepped sheet, flattening them into bagel shapes.
10. Sprinkle sesame seeds and bake for 30 minutes.

11. Remove oven and let them cool, enjoy!

Nutrition (Per Serving)

Total Carbs: 1.5g

Fiber: 1g

Protein: 2g

Fat: 5.8g

Nutmeg Nougats

Serving: 12

Prep Time: 10 minutes

Cooking Time: 5 minutes

Freeze Time: 30 minutes

Ingredients:

- 1 cup coconut, shredded

- 1 cup low-fat cream

- 1 cup cashew almond butter

- ½ teaspoon ground nutmeg

How To:

1. Melt the cashew almond butter over a double boiler.

2. Stir in nutmeg and dairy cream.
3. Remove from the heat.
4. Allow to cool down a little.
5. Keep in the refrigerator for at least 30 minutes.
6. Take out from the fridge and make small balls.
7. Coat with shredded coconut.

8.   Let it cool for 2 hours and then serve.

Nutrition (Per Serving)

Total Carbs: 13g

Fiber: 8g

Protein: 3g

Fat: 34g

Limey Savory Pie

Serving: 12

Prep Time: 5 minutes

Cooking Time: 5 minutes

Freeze Time: 2 hours

Ingredients:

- 1 tablespoon ground cinnamon

- 3 tablespoons almond butter

- 1 cup almond flour

- For the filling:

- 3 tablespoons grass-fed almond butter

- 4 ounces full-fat cream cheese

- ¼ cup coconut oil

- 2 limes

- A handful of baby spinach Stevia to taste

How To:

1.   Mix cinnamon and almond butter to form a crumble mixture.

2.   Press this mixture into the bottom of 12 muffin cups.
3.   Bake for 7 minutes at 350 degrees F.
4.   Juice the lime and grate for zest while the crust is baking.

5.   Take a food processor and add all the filling ingredients.

6.   Blend until smooth.
7.   Let it cool naturally.
8.   Pour the mixture in the center.
9.   Freeze until set and serve.

Nutrition (Per Serving)

Total Carbs: 2g

Fiber: 1g

Protein: 3g

Fat: 1g

Supreme Raspberry Chocolate Bombs

Serving: 6

Prep Time: 10 minutes

Cooking Time: 10 minutes

Freeze Time: 1-hour

Ingredients:

- ½ cacao almond butter

- ½ coconut manna

- 4 tablespoons powdered coconut almond milk

- 3 tablespoons granulated stevia

- ¼ cup dried and crushed raspberries, frozen

How To:

1.   Prepare your double boiler to medium heat and melt the cacao almond butter and coconut manna.

2.   Stir in vanilla extract.

3.   Take another dish and add coconut powder and sugar substitute.

4.   Stir the coconut mix into the cacao almond butter, 1 tablespoon at a time, making sure to keep mixing after each addition.
5.   Add the crushed dried raspberries.
6.   Mix well and portion it out into muffin tins.
7.   Chill for 60 minutes and enjoy!

Nutrition (Per Serving)

Total Carbs: 7g

Fiber: 1g

Protein: 11g

Fat: 21g

The Perfect Orange Ponzu

Serving: 8

Prep Time: 30 minutes

Cook Time: 5 minutes

Ingredients:

- ¼ cup coconut aminos

- ½ cup rice vinegar

- 2 tablespoons dry fish flakes

- 1 (1 inch) square kombu (kelp)

- 1 orange, quartered

How To:

1. Take a saucepan and place it over medium heat.

2. Add coconut aminos, rice vinegar, fish flakes, kombu, orange quarters and let the mixture sit for 30 minutes.
3. Bring the mix to a boil and immediately remove from the heat.

4. Let it cool and strain through a cheesecloth.

5. Serve and enjoy!

Nutrition (Per Serving)

Calories: 15

Fat: 0g

Carbohydrates: 4g

Protein: 0.8g

Hearty Cashew and Almond butter

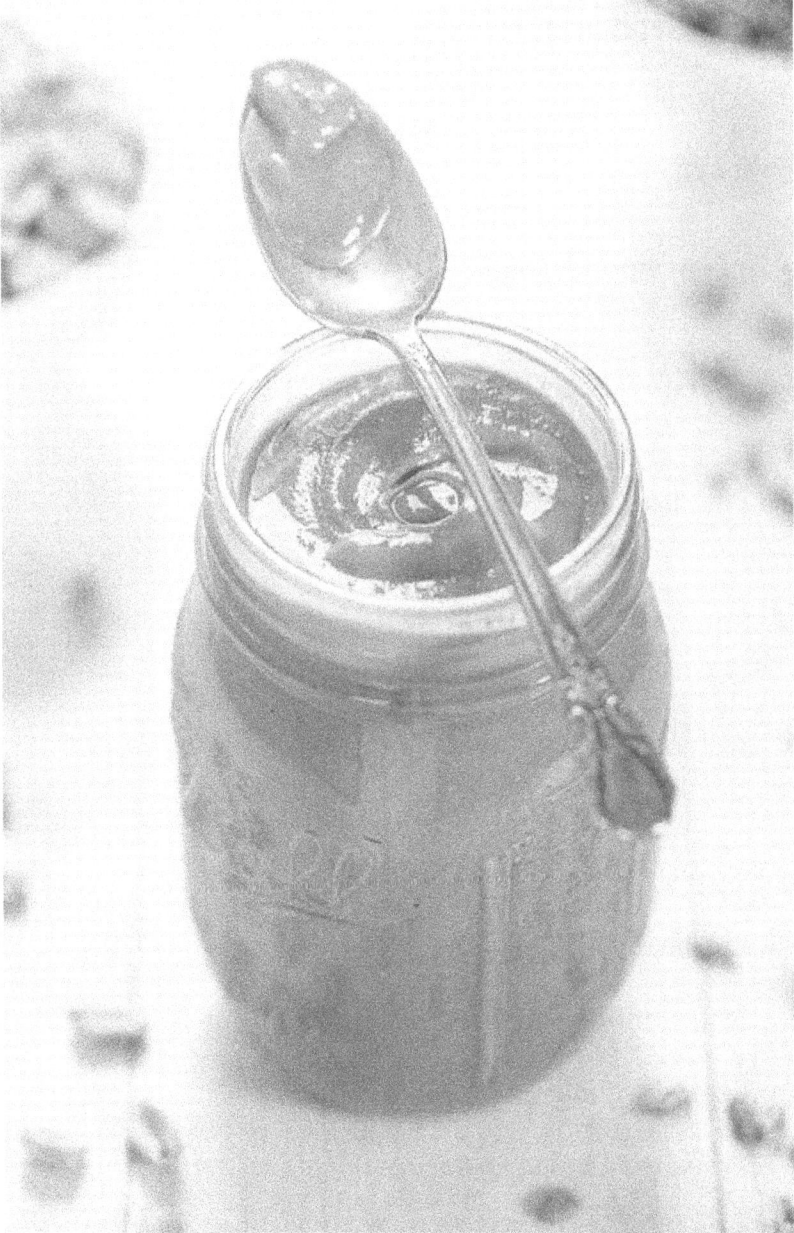

Serving: 1 and ½ cups

Prep Time: 5 minutes

Cook Time: Nil

Ingredients:

- 1 cup almonds, blanched

- 1/3 cup cashew nuts

- 2 tablespoons coconut oil

- Sunflower seeds as needed

- ½ teaspoon cinnamon

How To:

1. Pre-heat your oven to 350 degrees F.

2. Bake almonds and cashews for 12 minutes.

3. Let them cool.

4. Transfer to food processor and add remaining ingredients.

5. Add oil and keep blending until smooth.
6. Serve and enjoy! Nutrition (Per Serving)

Calories: 205

Fat: 19g

Carbohydrates: g[MOU3]

Protein: 2.8g

The Refreshing Nutter

Serving: 1

Prep Time: 10 minutes

Ingredients:

- 1 tablespoon chia seeds

- 2 cups water

- 1 ounces Macadamia Nuts

- 1-2 packets Stevia, optional

- 1 ounce hazelnut

How To:

1. Add all the listed ingredients to a blender.

2. Blend on high until smooth and creamy.
3. Enjoy your smoothie.

Nutrition (Per Serving)

Calories: 452

Fat: 43g

Carbohydrates: 15g

Protein: 9g

Elegant Cranberry Muffins

Serving: 24 muffins

Prep Time: 10 minutes

Cooking Time: 20 minutes

Ingredients:

- 2 cups almond flour

- 2 teaspoons baking soda

- ¼ cup avocado oil

- 1 whole egg

- ¾ cup almond milk

- ½ cup Erythritol

- ½ cup apple sauce

- Zest of 1 orange

- 2 teaspoons ground cinnamon

- 2 cup fresh cranberries

How To:

1.   Pre-heat your oven to 350 degrees F.

2.   Line muffin tin with paper muffin cups and keep them on the side.

3.   Add flour, baking soda and keep it on the side.
4.   Take another bowl and whisk in remaining ingredients and add flour, mix well.
5.   Pour batter into prepared muffin tin and bake for 20 minutes.
6.   Once done, let it cool for 10 minutes.
7.   Serve and enjoy!

Nutrition (Per Serving)

Total Carbs: 7g

Fiber: 2g

Protein: 2.3g

Fat: 7g

Apple and Almond Muffins

Serving: 6 muffins

Prep Time: 10 minutes

Cooking Time: 20 minutes

Ingredients:

- 6 ounces ground almonds

- 1 teaspoon cinnamon

- ½ teaspoon baking powder

- 1 pinch sunflower seed

- 1 whole egg

- 1 teaspoon apple cider vinegar

- 2 tablespoons Erythritol

- 1/3 cup apple sauce

How To:

1.   Pre-heat your oven to 350 degrees F.

2.   Line muffin tin with paper muffin cups, keep them on the side.

3.   Mix in almonds, cinnamon, baking powder, sunflower seeds and keep it on the side.
4.   Take another bowl and beat in eggs, apple cider vinegar, apple sauce, Erythritol.
5.   Add the mix to dry ingredients and mix well until you have a smooth batter.
6.   Pour batter into tin and bake for 20 minutes.
7.   Once done, let them cool.
8.   Serve and enjoy!

Nutrition (Per Serving)

Total Carbs: 10

Fiber: 4g

Protein: 13g

Fat: 17g

Stylish Chocolate Parfait

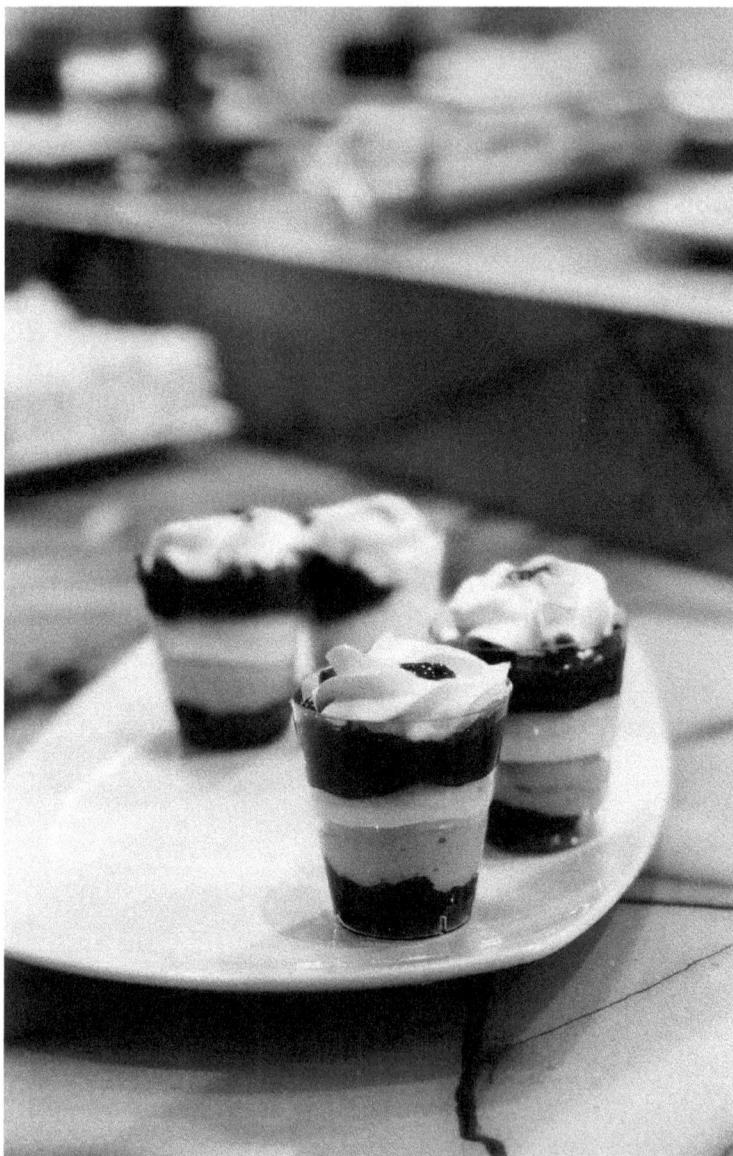

Serving: 4

Prep Time: 2 hours

Cook Time: nil

Ingredients:

- 2 tablespoons cocoa powder `
- 1 cup almond milk
- 1 tablespoon chia seeds
- Pinch of sunflower seeds
- ½ teaspoon vanilla extract

How To:

1. Take a bowl and add cocoa powder, almond milk, chia seeds, vanilla extract and stir.

2. Transfer to dessert glass and place in your fridge for 2 hours.
3. Serve and enjoy!

Nutrition (Per Serving)

Calories: 130

Fat: 5g

Carbohydrates: 7g

Protein: 16g

Supreme Matcha Bomb

Serving: 10

Prep Time: 100 minutes

Cook Time: Nil

Ingredients:

- 3/4 cup hemp seeds

- ½ cup coconut oil

- 2 tablespoons coconut almond butter

- 1 teaspoon Matcha powder

- 2 tablespoons vanilla bean extract

- ½ teaspoon mint extract Liquid stevia

How To:

1.   Take your blender/food processor and add hemp seeds, coconut oil, Matcha, vanilla extract and stevia.

2.   Blend until you have a nice batter and divide into silicon molds.

3.   Melt coconut almond butter and drizzle on top.

4.   Let the cups chill and enjoy!

Nutrition (Per Serving)
Calories: 200

Fat: 20g

Carbohydrates: 3g

Protein: 5g

Mesmerizing Avocado and Chocolate Pudding

Serving: 2

Prep Time: 30 minutes

Cook Time: Nil

Ingredients:

1 avocado, chunked

- 1 tablespoon natural sweetener such as stevia

- 2 ounces cream cheese, at room temp

- ¼ teaspoon vanilla extract

- 4 tablespoons cocoa powder, unsweetened

How To:

1. Blend listed ingredients in blender until smooth.

2. Divide the mix between dessert bowls, chill for 30 minutes.

3. Serve and enjoy!

Nutrition (Per Serving)

Calories: 281

Fat: 27g

Carbohydrates: 12g

Protein: 8g

Hearty Pineapple Pudding

Serving: 4

Prep Time: 10 minutes

Cooking Time: 5 hours

Ingredients:

- 1 teaspoon baking powder

- 1 cup coconut flour

- 3 tablespoons stevia

- 3 tablespoons avocado oil

- ½ cup coconut milk

- ½ cup pecans, chopped

- ½ cup pineapple, chopped

- ½ cup lemon zest, grated

- 1 cup pineapple juice, natural

How To:

1.   Grease Slow Cooker with oil.

2.   Take a bowl and mix in flour, stevia, baking powder, oil, milk, pecans, pineapple, lemon zest, pineapple juice and stir well.
3.   Pour the mix into the Slow Cooker.
4.   Place lid and cook on LOW for 5 hours.
5.   Divide between bowls and serve.
6.   Enjoy!

Nutrition (Per Serving)

Calories: 188

Fat: 3g

Carbohydrates: 14g

Protein: 5g

Healthy Berry Cobbler

Serving: 8

Prep Time: 10 minutes

Cooking Time: 2 hours 30 minutes

Ingredients:

- 1 ¼ cups almond flour

- 1 cup coconut sugar

- 1 teaspoon baking powder

- ½ teaspoon cinnamon powder

- 1 whole egg

- ¼ cup low-fat milk

- 2 tablespoons olive oil

- 2 cups raspberries

- 2 cups blueberries

How To:

1.   Take a bowl and add almond flour, coconut sugar, baking powder and cinnamon.

2.   Stir well .
3.   Take another bowl and add egg, milk, oil, raspberries, blueberries and stir.
4.   Combine both of the mixtures.
5.   Grease your Slow Cooker.
6.   Pour the combined mixture into your Slow Cooker and cook on HIGH for 2 hours 30 minutes.   ·
7.   Divide between serving bowls and enjoy!

Nutrition (Per Serving)

Calories: 250

Fat: 4g

Carbohydrates: 30g

Protein: 3g

Tasty Poached Apples

Serving: 8

Prep Time: 10 minutes

Cooking Time: 2 hours 30 minutes

Ingredients:

- 6 apples, cored, peeled and sliced

- 1 cup apple juice, natural

- 1 cup coconut sugar

- 1 tablespoon cinnamon powder

How To:

1.   Grease Slow Cooker with cooking spray.

2.   Add apples, sugar, juice, cinnamon to your Slow Cooker.
3.   Stir gently.
4.   Place lid and cook on HIGH for 4 hours.
5.   Serve cold and enjoy!

Nutrition (Per Serving)

Calories: 180

Fat: 5g

Carbohydrates: 8g

Protein: 4g

Home Made Trail Mix For The Trip

Serving: 4

Prep Time: 10 minutes

Cook Time: 55 minutes

Ingredients:

- ¼ cup raw cashews

- ¼ cup almonds

- ¼ cup walnuts

- 1 teaspoon cinnamon

- 2 tablespoons melted coconut oil

- Sunflower seeds as needed

How To:

1.   Line baking sheet with parchment paper.

2.   Pre-heat your oven to 275 degrees F.

3.   Melt coconut oil and keep it on the side.
4.   Combine nuts to large mixing bowl and add cinnamon and melted coconut oil.

5.   Stir.
6.   Sprinkle sunflower seeds.
7.   Place in oven and brown for 6 minutes.
8.   Enjoy!

Nutrition (Per Serving)

Calories: 363

Fat: 22g

Carbohydrates: 41g

Protein: 7g

Heart Warming Cinnamon Rice Pudding

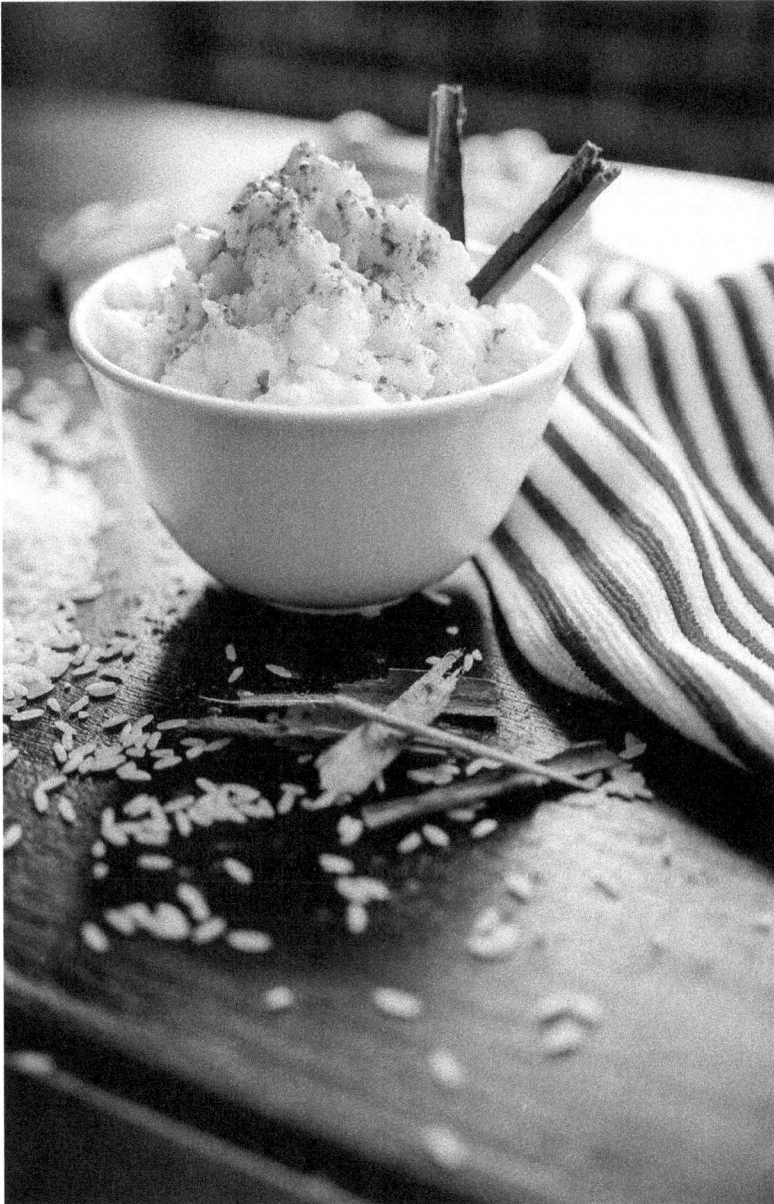

Serving: 4

Prep Time: 10 minutes

Cooking Time: 5 hours

Ingredients:

- 6 ½ cups water

- 1 cup coconut sugar

- 2 cups white rice

- 2 cinnamon sticks

- ½ cup coconut, shredded

How To:

1.   Add water, rice, sugar, cinnamon and coconut to your Slow Cooker.

2.   Gently stir.
3.   Place lid and cook on HIGH for 5 hours.
4.   Discard cinnamon.
5.   Divide pudding between dessert dishes and enjoy!
Nutrition (Per Serving)

Calories: 173

Fat: 4g

Carbohydrates: 9g

Protein: 4g

Pure Avocado Pudding

Serving: 4

Prep Time: 3 hours

Cook Time: nil

Ingredients:

1 cup almond milk

- 2 avocados, peeled and pitted

- ¾ cup cocoa powder

- 1 teaspoon vanilla extract

- 2 tablespoons stevia

- ¼ teaspoon cinnamon

- Walnuts, chopped for serving

How To:

1.   Add avocados to a blender and pulse well.

2.   Add cocoa powder, almond milk, stevia, vanilla bean extract and pulse the mixture well.
3.   Pour into serving bowls and top with walnuts.
4.   Chill for 2-3 hours and serve!

Nutrition (Per Serving)

Calories: 221

Fat: 8g

Carbohydrates: 7g

Protein: 3g

Sweet Almond and Coconut Fat Bombs

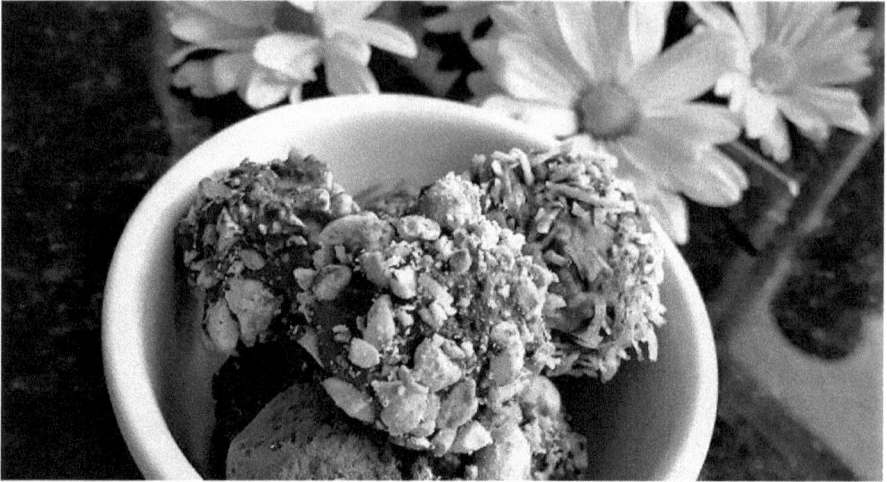

Serving: 6

Prep Time: 10 minutes

Cooking Time: 10 minutes

Freeze Time: 20 minutes

Ingredients:

- ¼ cup melted coconut oil

- 9 ½ tablespoons almond butter

- 90 drops liquid stevia

- 3 tablespoons cocoa

- 9 tablespoons melted almond butter, sunflower seeds

How To:

1.   Take a bowl and add all of the listed ingredients.

2.   Mix them well.
3.   Pour 2 tablespoons of the mixture into as many muffin molds as you like.
4.   Chill for 20 minutes and pop them out.
5.   Serve and enjoy!

Nutrition (Per Serving)

Total Carbs: 2g

Fiber: 0g

Protein: 2.53g

Fat: 14g

Spicy Popper Mug Cake

Serving: 2

Prep Time: 5 minutes

Cook Time: 5 minutes

Ingredients:

- 2 tablespoons almond flour

- 1 tablespoon flaxseed meal

- 1 tablespoon almond butter

- 1 tablespoon cream cheese

- 1 large egg

- 1 bacon, cooked and sliced

- ½ jalapeno pepper

- ½ teaspoon baking powder

¼ teaspoon sunflower seeds

How To:

1.   Take a frying pan and place it over medium heat.

2.   Add slice of bacon and cook until it has a crispy texture.
3.   Take a microwave proof container and mix all of the listed ingredients (including cooked bacon), clean the sides.
4.   Microwave for 75 seconds, making to put your microwave to high power.
5.   Take out the cup and tap it against a surface to take the cake out.

6.   Garnish with a bit of jalapeno and serve!

Nutrition (Per Serving)

Calories: 429

Fat: 38g

Carbohydrates: 6g

Protein: 16g

The Most Elegant Parsley Soufflé Ever

Serving: 5

Prep Time: 5 minutes

Cook Time: 6 minutes

Ingredients:

- 2 whole eggs

- 1 fresh red chili pepper, chopped

- 2 tablespoons coconut cream

- 1 tablespoon fresh parsley, chopped Sunflower seeds to taste

How To:

1. Pre-heat your oven to 390 degrees F.

2.   Almond butter 2 soufflé dishes.

3.   Add the ingredients to a blender and mix well.
4.   Divide batter into soufflé dishes and bake for 6 minutes.
5.   Serve and enjoy!

Nutrition (Per Serving)

Calories: 108

Fat: 9g

Carbohydrates: 9g

Protein: 6g

Fennel and Almond Bites

Serving: 12

Prep Time: 10 minutes

Cooking Time: None

Freeze Time: 3 hours

Ingredients:

- 1 teaspoon vanilla extract

- ¼ cup almond milk

- ¼ cup cocoa powder

- ½ cup almond oil

- A pinch of sunflower seeds

- 1 teaspoon fennel seeds

How To:

1.   Take a bowl and mix the almond oil and almond milk.

2.   Beat until smooth and glossy using electric beater.
3.   Mix in the rest of the ingredients.
4.   Take a piping bag and pour into a parchment paper lined baking sheet.
5.   Freeze for 3 hours and store in the fridge.

Nutrition (Per Serving)

Total Carbs: 1g

Fiber: 1g

Protein: 1g

Fat: 20g

Feisty Coconut Fudge

Serving: 12

Prep Time: 20 minutes

Cooking Time: None

Freeze Time: 2 hours

Ingredients:

- ¼ cup coconut, shredded

- 2 cups coconut oil

- ½ cup coconut cream

- ¼ cup almonds, chopped

- 1 teaspoon almond extract

- A pinch of sunflower seeds

- Stevia to taste

How To:

1.   Take a large bowl and pour coconut cream and coconut oil into it.

2.   Whisk using an electric beater.
3.   Whisk until the mixture becomes smooth and glossy.
4.   Add cocoa powder slowly and mix well.
5.   Add in the rest of the ingredients.
6.   Pour into a bread pan lined with parchment paper.
7.   Freeze until set.
8.   Cut them into squares and serve.

Nutrition (Per Serving)

Total Carbs: 1g

Fiber: 1g

Protein: 0g

Fat: 20g

No Bake Cheesecake

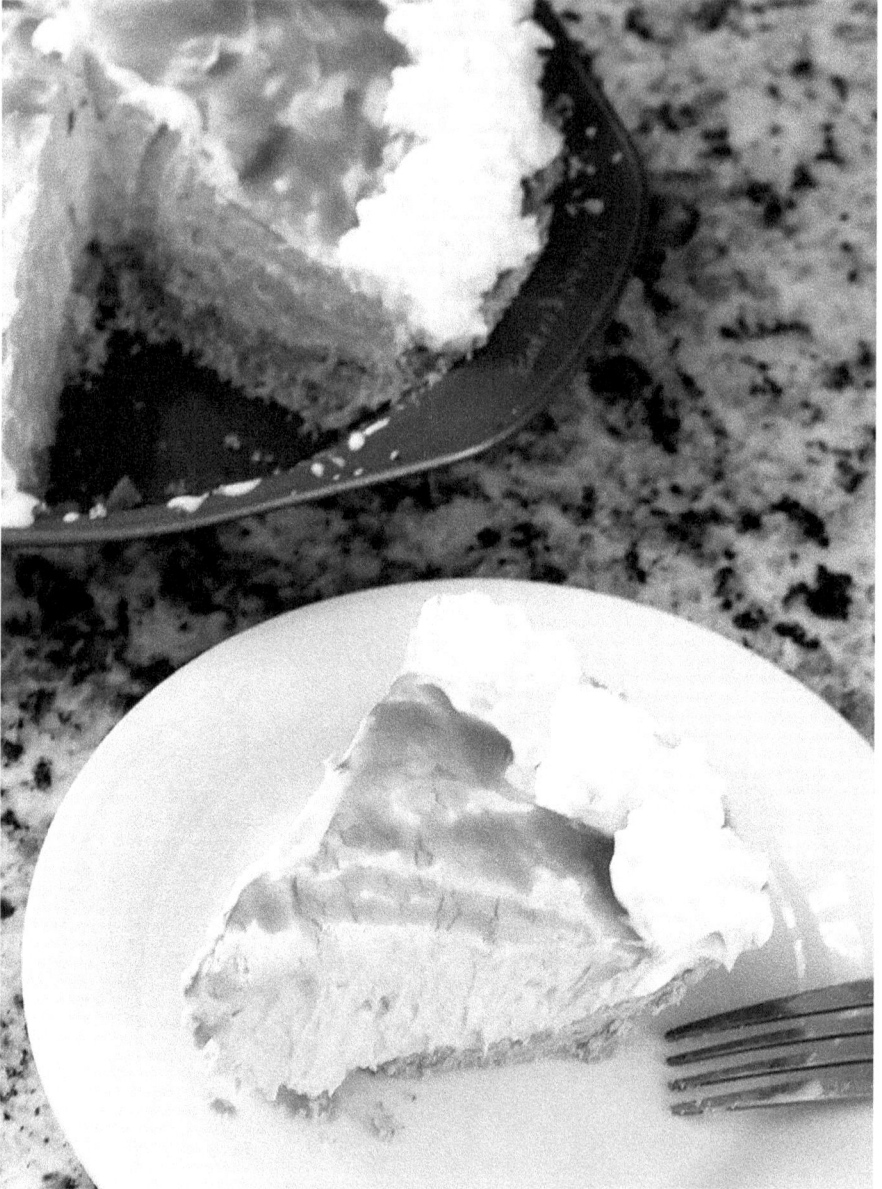

Serving: 10

Prep Time: 120 minutes

Cook Time: Nil

Ingredients:

For Crust

- 2 tablespoons ground flaxseeds

- 2 tablespoons desiccated coconut

- 1 teaspoon cinnamon

For Filling

- 4 ounces vegan cream cheese

- 1 cup cashews, soaked

- ½ cup frozen blueberries

- 2 tablespoons coconut oil

- 1 tablespoon lemon juice

- 1 teaspoon vanilla extract Liquid stevia

How To:

1.   Take a container and mix in the crust ingredients, mix well.

2.   Flatten the mixture at the bottom to prepare the crust of your cheesecake.
3.   Take a blender/ food processor and add the filling ingredients, blend until smooth.
4.   Gently pour the batter on top of your crust and chill for 2 hours.

5.   Serve and enjoy!

Nutrition (Per Serving)

Calories: 182

Fat: 16g

Carbohydrates: 4g

Protein: 3g

Easy Chia Seed Pumpkin Pudding

Serving: 4

Prep Time: 10-15 minutes/ overnight chill time

Cook Time: Nil

Ingredients:

- 1 cup maple syrup

- 2 teaspoons pumpkin spice

- 1 cup pumpkin puree

- 1 ¼ cup almond milk

- ½ cup chia seeds

How To:

1.   Add all of the ingredients to a bowl and gently stir.

2.   Let it refrigerate overnight or at least 15 minutes.
3.   Top with your desired ingredients, such as blueberries, almonds, etc.
4.   Serve and enjoy!

Nutrition (Per Serving)

Calories: 230

Fat: 10g

Carbohydrates:22g

Protein:11g

Lovely Blueberry Pudding

Serving: 4

Prep Time: 20 minutes

Cook Time: Nil

Ingredients:

- 2 cups frozen blueberries

- 2 teaspoons lime zest, grated freshly

- 20 drops liquid stevia

- 2 small avocados, peeled, pitted and chopped

- ½ teaspoon fresh ginger, grated freshly

- 4 tablespoons fresh lime juice

- 10 tablespoons water

How To:

1.   Add all of the listed ingredients to a blender (except blueberries) and pulse the mixture well.

2.   Transfer the mix into small serving bowls and chill the bowls.
3.   Serve with a topping of blueberries.
4.   Enjoy!

Nutrition (Per Serving)

Calories: 166

Fat: 13g

Carbohydrates: 13g

Protein: 1.7g

Decisive Lime and Strawberry Popsicle

Serving: 4

Prep Time: 2 hours

Cook Time: Nil

Ingredients:

- 1 tablespoon lime juice, fresh

- ¼ cup strawberries, hulled and sliced

- ¼ cup coconut almond milk, unsweetened and full fat

- 2 teaspoons natural sweetener

How To:

1.   Blend the listed ingredients in a blender until smooth.

2.   Pour mix into popsicle molds and let them chill for 2 hours.
3.   Serve and enjoy!

Nutrition (Per Serving)

Calories: 166

Fat: 17g

Carbohydrates: 3g

Protein: 1g